POWER
CRYSTALS
JOURNAL

© 2014 Fair Winds Press
Text © 2011 Judy Hall

First published in the USA in 2014 by
Fair Winds Press, a member of
Quayside Publishing Group
100 Cummings Center
Suite 406-L
Beverly, MA 01915-6101
www.fairwindspress.com

18 17 16 15 14   1 2 3 4 5

ISBN: 978-1-59233-627-2

Cover image: Trigonic Quartz
Original book design by Kathie Alexander
Journal design by Laura H. Couallier, Laura Herrmann Design
Photography by Exquisite Crystals, www.exquisitecrystals.com

Printed and bound in China

The information in this book is for educational purposes only. It is not intended to
replace the advice of a physician or medical practitioner. Please see your health care
provider before beginning any new health program.

POWER CRYSTALS JOURNAL

A Guided Journal to Magical Crystals, Gems, and Stones for Healing and Transformation

JUDY HALL

C rystals have always been regarded as a source of power—and as a gift from the gods. Impressive no matter what their size, gems hold an aura of mystery and authority. From prehistory to the present, gemstones have symbolized wealth and been accorded wondrous properties. The ancient texts that tell us so much about the power of stones had their origins in the Stone Age, a time when technology quite literally came from stones. Since that time, we have continued to harness their magical power.

This journal can serve as a record of your use of crystals. Include everything you experienced—sights, sounds, tactile experiences, tastes, scents. Write the "story" of what happened. Most important, write how you benefited from the experience. Feel it as you write it.

Right Use of Power

Crystals work by cooperating with you to focus and manifest your intention. Be clear about why you are working with the crystal and ensure that you are working for the highest good. Misuse of crystal power will inevitably rebound. Like humans, crystals can become exhausted, so re-empowering them regularly is a sensible precaution. As crystals rapidly draw off energy from their surroundings, they need purifying at frequent intervals.

Purifying Your Crystals

Crystals pick up energy from anyone who handles them and from the environment, so they need cleansing before and after use. Purify a crystal by holding it under running water—so long as the crystal won't dissolve or fragment. Then put it in the sun or moonlight to reenergize it. You can also smudge a crystal with incense smoke, place it in candlelight, or leave it overnight in uncooked brown rice.

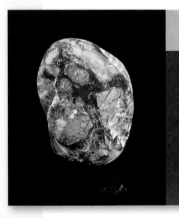

CRYSTAL ATTUNEMENT

Take a few moments to attune to a crystal. Hold a purified crystal in your hands and feel its vibrations radiating into your being. If they are in accord with your own, you will feel calm, peaceful, and quite possibly expanded. If you feel uncomfortable, choose another stone—the one you are holding might not be right for you at this time, or may indicate you have inner work to do.

Activating the Power of Your Crystal

To activate your crystal's power, hold the purified crystal in your hands, focus your intention and attention on it, and say: "I dedicate this crystal to the highest good of all and ask that its power be activated now to work in harmony with my own will and focused intention."

If you have a specific purpose, add that to your dedication. To deactivate the crystal, cleanse it and then hold the crystal as you say: "I thank this crystal for its power, which is no longer needed at this time. I ask that its power be closed until reactivated."

Put the crystal in the sun to recharge it, and then place it in a bag, box, or a drawer until it is required again. If you are placing crystals in a grid, layout for cleaning, or to create safe space, join up the shape either by touching each stone with a crystal wand or by using the power of your mind to picture lines of light connecting the stones and making the shape.

Using Your Crystal Power

After you have empowered your crystal, you can wear it daily, preferably in contact with your skin. Or, place it on your body or in your environment to radiate out or draw on the power as appropriate. A piece of Black Tourmaline or Amber, for instance, placed in each corner of your home invokes the power of protection and energy screening, safeguarding you. Or, you can use your crystal for healing or to expand your consciousness.

To expand your consciousness with high-vibration crystals, either place a crystal on your third eye, soma, or higher crown chakra, or sit holding the stone. Breathe gently and focus your awareness on the crystal. Do not try to see or experience anything, simply let the process unfold. Notice any changes, without giving them undue attention.

After ten to twenty minutes (no longer), remove the crystal. Picture yourself totally surrounded by a bubble of crystal light. Feel the contact your feet make with the Earth, and then get up and go about your everyday business. If you feel "floaty" or unfocused, hold a Smoky Quartz or Hematite as you visualize roots growing from the balls of your feet, joining at the earth star chakra, and then going down into the center of the Earth where they attach to the ball of iron at its center to create a shamanic anchor.

Agate

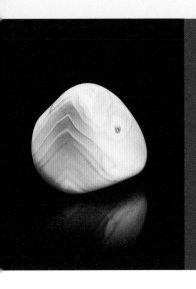

HARNESSING THE POWER

Wear Agate or keep one in your pocket and touch it frequently to give you strength.

TRANSFORMATIONAL POWER

Agate puts you in touch with your inner self. Its power lies in its ability to transmute dark, toxic emotions such as jealousy, bitterness, and resentment, which have a psychosomatic effect on the body, creating dis-ease in the heart and unrest in the soul. Due to its powerful cleansing effect, Agate helps you assimilate challenging life experiences and recognize the spiritual gifts they offer. By promoting self-acceptance and forgiveness, Agate increases receptivity to spiritual currents in your life. Carrying an Agate stimulates courage to start again and encourages you to hold fast to your own truth. It helps you recognize your eternal nature and the oneness of all things.

Travelers in the Arabian and African deserts sucked Agates to overcome the effects of thirst.

AGATE

Amazonite

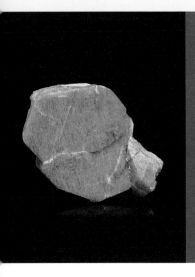

HARNESSING THE POWER

To share the power of friendship, give your friends Amazonites. Schedule a regular time when you will think of each other while holding your stones.

_____

_____

_____

_____

_____

_____

_____

_____

_____

_____

_____

_____

_____

*Amazonite shields
the body from
the effects of subtle
radiation and
electromagnetic
frequencies
including Wi-Fi.*

AMAZONITE

Amber

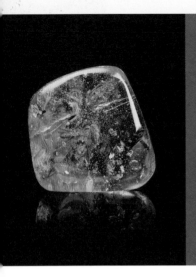

HARNESSING THE POWER

Hold a piece of Amber above your head and imagine it slowly melting, pouring a protective coating around your aura to seal it.

TRANSFORMATIONAL POWER

Amber can be used to transmute negative vibrations into positive ones. It creates an efficient screen against negative energies of all kinds. Placed on the body, it energetically cleanses and reactivates the chakras and your psychic immune system. Put Amber in the corners of a sickroom to keep it energetically clean and to shield the patient against adverse environmental energies.

Amber ignites easily, and the ancients believed its smoke drove away evil spirits and enchantments, as well as relieving sinus and respiratory ailments and throat infections.

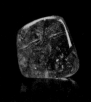

AMBER

Amethyst

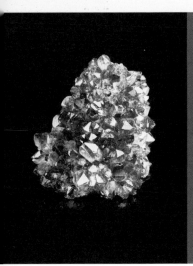

HARNESSING THE POWER

Place an Amethyst above your head, point toward you, and one on your forehead, pointing down. Feel peace radiating through your body.

TRANSFORMATIONAL POWER

Amethyst opens your third eye and clarifies spiritual vision. By creating a safe sacred space for meditation and multidimensional exploration, it clears your mind and aids enlightenment. High-vibration Amethysts, such as Vera Cruz, act on an altogether different level. Placed on the soul star or stellar gateway chakra, they stimulate your soul to remember its origins and facilitate multidimensional cellular healing. By detaching you from unwanted entities, thought forms, or mental constructs, Amethyst dispels illusions that prevent you from experiencing true reality. It helps you dream a new world into being.

Traditionally, Amethyst was bound to the forehead to heal headaches, and modern-day crystal workers use Amethyst to calm anxiety and draw off physical or psychological pain.

AMETHYST

Black Tourmaline (Schorl)

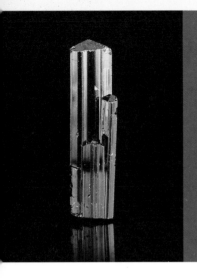

HARNESSING THE POWER

To instantly stop jealousy,
ill will, or all-out psychic attack,
wear Black Tourmaline over
your thymus. The stone safely
defuses the attack.

TRANSFORMATIONAL POWER

Black Tourmaline is invaluable for sensitive people who are overwhelmed by geopathic or electromagnetic stress, including Wi-Fi, or by radiation. It draws the toxicity out through your feet and transmutes it into powerful Earth-healing energy. Wear Black Tourmaline at your throat or place it on your computer or other electrical equipment to block emanations and strengthen your auric field.

Most Black Tourmaline contains iron, making it a powerfully protective stone.

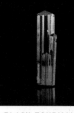

BLACK TOURMALINE
(SCHORL)

Bronzite

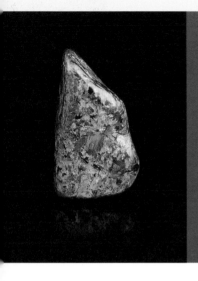

HARNESSING THE POWER

To create a safe, sacred space
for meditation, lay out tumbled
Bronzites to form a six-pointed star
with a stone at each point.

TRANSFORMATIONAL POWER

Bronzite's strong magnetic flow provides an inner compass to assist in finding your direction: physically and spiritually. If you tend to judge other people or yourself harshly, Bronzite teaches the power of compassion and forgiveness. If you feel powerless in a situation or have handed your power over to someone else, holding Bronzite calls your power back and helps you take the course of right action. Conversely, if you have been overly willful, especially in past lives, Bronzite teaches you to attune your will so you are guided by your soul rather than your ego.

Sold as a magical protector, Bronzite must be used with care because it may amplify and exacerbate the effects of ill intent, spells, and psychic attack.

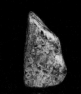

BRONZITE

Carnelian

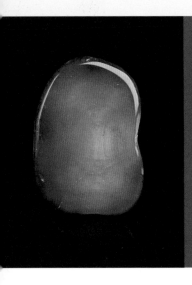

HARNESSING THE POWER

Place a Carnelian where you will
see it often. Each time you pass
the stone, touch it and say,
"I am grateful."

_____

_____

_____

_____

_____

_____

_____

_____

_____

_____

_____

*Modern crystal
workers prize
Carnelian for its
ability to energize.
It may benefit
infertility, impotence,
and frigidity.*

CARNELIAN

Cathedral Quartz

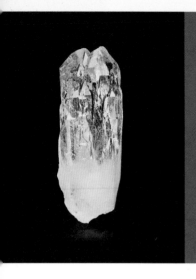

HARNESSING THE POWER

Meditate with Cathedral Quartz daily to raise the frequency of your mind, encouraging positive thought and intention.

*Cathedral Quartz
has the master
healing power of
Quartz taken to
a higher dimension,
to work on cellular
memory from the
vibration of light.*

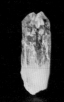

CATHEDRAL
QUARTZ

Diamond

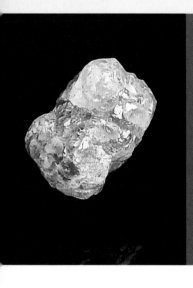

HARNESSING THE POWER

Wear a Diamond, the traditional
gem for engagement rings,
to ensure eternal harmony
between lovers.

TRANSFORMATIONAL POWER

A Diamond is dull until faceted
and polished; its beauty and
brilliance must be revealed slowly
with patience and care.
The cut is crucial for the finished
gemstone's perfection. Unaffected
by fire's heat or water's coolness,
it symbolizes magical survival
through elemental changes.
Wearing this crystal provides
protection and assists in the
assimilation of expanded
consciousness and soul evolution.

Diamond acts at the mental level to induce clarity and stimulate imagination.
It protects against geopathic stress and electromagnetic frequencies.

DIAMOND

THE POWER OF INTEGRATION
Elestial Quartz

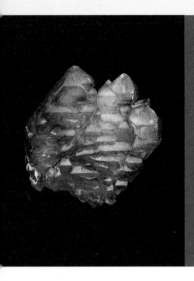

HARNESSING THE POWER

Hold Elestial to understand the breadth of your soul and its experiences and to recognize that inner work, not words or deeds, propels spiritual evolution.

_____

_____

_____

_____

_____

_____

_____

_____

_____

_____

_____

_____

_____

_____

TRANSFORMATIONAL POWER

The finest transmutor of negative energy, Smoky Elestial grounds grids into everyday reality and anchors healings for the body or Earth. It pulls negative energy out of the environment, transmutes it, and protects the area. In karmic healing, Smoky Elestial helps to reframe the etheric blueprint and ancestral line, transmuting energy back to the beginning of that line so the cellular memory is reprogrammed and power is restored to future generations.

Elestial Quartz rapidly expands your spiritual evolution, preparing the light and physical bodies and stabilizing energy shifts.

ELESTIAL QUARTZ

Emerald

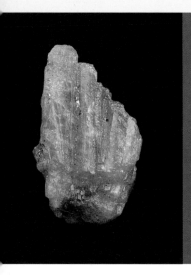

HARNESSING THE POWER

Wear Emerald to attract successful love—and keep it once you have found it. This stone has long been believed to ensure a happy marriage.

TRANSFORMATIONAL POWER

Emerald symbolizes immortality and rebirth. Whether raw or faceted, this stone provides enormous inspiration on the spiritual path and gives you patience to pass through challenges with equanimity. Promoting friendship and unconditional love, Emerald enhances relationships on all levels, keeping partnerships in harmony. The stone balances the emotional, mental, and spiritual levels, transmuting negativity into positive action. It has long been used to stimulate metaphysical abilities, opening a broader vision that sees beyond the projections of the material world.

The ancient Greek philosopher Theophrastus tells us Emerald was good for eyes, imparting visual clarity.

EMERALD

Fluorite

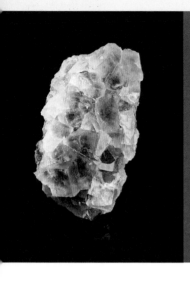

HARNESSING THE POWER

If you need more stability in your life, mind, body, or emotions, carry Fluorite at all times to give you inner strength.

Fluorite helps disorganized people to think straight and get their lives back on track. If you are under any illusions, Fluorite dissolves them so that you can make objective decisions.

Regarded as a natural antiviral, immune stimulator, and anti-inflammatory agent, Fluorite restores order to the body, particularly the lungs and bones.

FLUORITE

Garnet

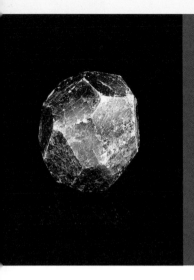

HARNESSING THE POWER

Carry Garnet when it seems you
will never achieve your goal.
It brings hope and the power to
succeed in hopeless situations.

TRANSFORMATIONAL POWER

Wearing Garnet helps you be faithful to a partner while remaining true to yourself. In ancient times, rounded red Garnets were known as carbuncles, reminding us that they draw festering emotions to the surface for transmutation. With the stone's assistance, you can convert pain, resentment, and dis-ease into well-being. Garnet lets you recognize where you may be sabotaging yourself or resisting change, and it gives you the courage to speak out plus the stamina to maintain your transformation. With Garnet's assistance, you can remain faithful to your purpose.

In medieval times,
Garnets were famed
for their curative and
protective powers,
and used to
neutralize poison,
reduce depression,
and calm fever.

GARNET

Granite

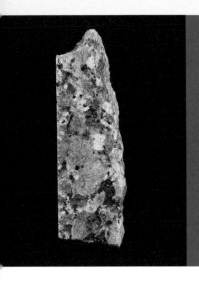

HARNESSING THE POWER

Place a piece of Granite on the floor at each corner of your bed to boost the flow of energy through your body.

TRANSFORMATIONAL POWER

Egyptologist Robert Bauval has described human beings as "star material become conscious" because our bodies contain minerals and elements from outer space. The ancient Egyptians knew about Granite's ability to transform the human energy field to a higher resonance and encouraged humankind to look to the stars for their origins. They utilized Granite to draw the power of the gods to Earth and to assist the Pharaoh on his shamanic journey to the stars.

Granite grids can neutralize the ill effects of toxic Earth energy lines and reenergize the Earth's magnetic matrix.

GRANITE

Hematite

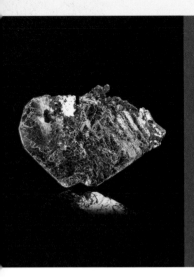

HARNESSING THE POWER

Carry Hematite in your pocket
to create a power shield that
protects you from electromagnetic
smog and geopathic, physical,
or mental stress.

According to Greek myth, Hematite was created when Saturn killed his father, the tyrannical god Uranus. This ancient "cycle myth" describes the destruction of the old to make way for the new.

HEMATITE

Jade

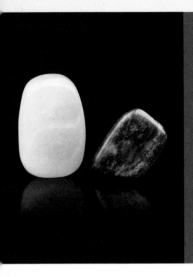

HARNESSING THE POWER

Hold Jade over your solar plexus
for a few minutes each day to
stabilize your psyche and emotions
and help you live harmoniously
on the Earth.

The Chinese considered Jade the most precious gem as it held five great virtues—wisdom, justice, modesty, courage, and purity—plus five happinesses—wealth, old age, health, natural death, and love of virtue.

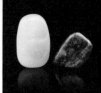

JADE

Moldavite

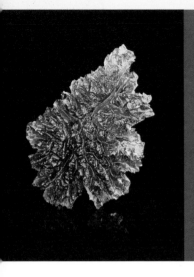

HARNESSING THE POWER

Meditate with Moldavite on your third eye to connect to the highest planes of consciousness and become one with the cosmos.

TRANSFORMATIONAL POWER

A crystal of karmic and soul transformation, Moldavite downloads information from the Akashic Record and instills cosmic consciousness. It takes you back into your past to reconnect to your previous wisdom and soul purpose, and into the future to access what you need for your soul's evolution. Then it lets you put that knowledge into practice in the present. (Note: if you are sensitive or unaccustomed to high-vibration crystals, wear or use Moldavite sparingly until an energetic adjustment is made.)

*More than
twenty-five thousand
years ago, the people
of Eastern Europe
used Moldavite
as a talisman to
enhance fertility
and good fortune
and fashioned tools
from it.*

MOLDAVITE

Nirvana Quartz

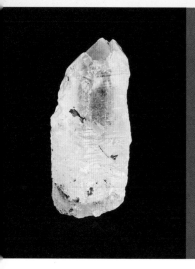

HARNESSING THE POWER

Meditate with Nirvana Quartz
to induce a bliss-like state of
unconditional love combined with
pure mind in which the divine
infuses the physical realm.

Nirvana is one of the highest vibration Quartzes yet discovered. A crystal of spiritual alchemy, it attunes the flame of pure consciousness to the soul star chakra so that the light of expansion and enlightenment flows through the body and into the Earth.

NIRVANA QUARTZ

Obsidian

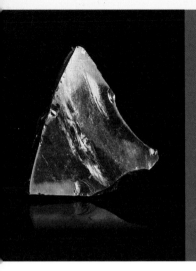

HARNESSING THE POWER

Place Obsidian at your feet.
Visualize cords passing from each
foot, going through the earth star,
entwining deep into the Earth,
anchoring you during turmoil.

At a physical level, Obsidian draws off negativity, assisting the body's structures to energetically detoxify, soften, and realign.

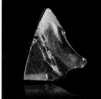

OBSIDIAN

Opal

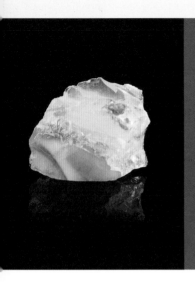

HARNESSING THE POWER

Hold your Opal, focus your attention into the crystal, and visualize what you wish to manifest. It will come into being.

In Greco-Roman times, Opal was associated with Hermes/Mercury, who conveyed the souls of the dead to the underworld.

OPAL

Paraiba Tourmaline

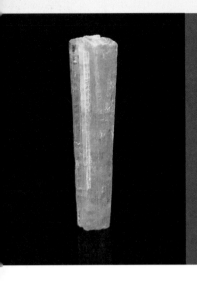

HARNESSING THE POWER

Place Paraiba Tourmaline over the past life chakra for a few minutes each day to bring unfinished business to its natural conclusion.

TRANSFORMATIONAL POWER

Paraiba works its magical trans-
formations on several levels.
A stone of compassionate being,
it stimulates the radiant heart,
opening the heart seed chakra and
bringing unconditional love into
the Earth plane. It teaches you how
to love yourself and others from the
soul's perspective. Stimulating
spiritual evolution by opening the
stellar gateway, it identifies where
you have strayed from your truth,
bringing you back to the path
of awareness and facilitating
expression of your true feelings.
If outdated, ingrained beliefs,
karmic wounds, or mental
constructs are blocking the
way, Paraiba gently dissolves
them and helps you forgive
yourself and others.

Paraiba works mostly at the emotional and spiritual levels, encouraging forgiveness and releasing bitterness in the heart.

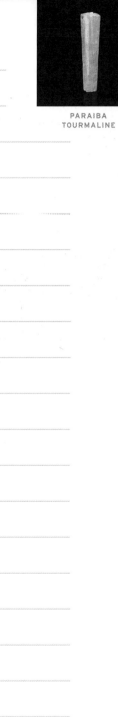

PARAIBA
TOURMALINE

Poppy Jasper

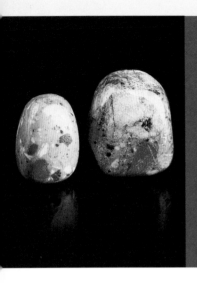

HARNESSING THE POWER

Kept in your pocket or under your pillow, Poppy Jasper speeds recovery during illness, convalescence, or hospitalization.

Poppy Jasper's red
spots within the
colorful Jasper matrix
give it the appearance
of a field of poppies.

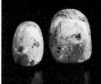

POPPY JASPER

Quartz

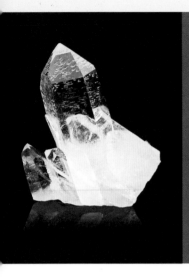

HARNESSING THE POWER

Place Quartz wherever healing is needed. It restores your whole being to energetic harmony and wholeness.

TRANSFORMATIONAL POWER

Quartz holds a dynamic hologram of the soul and universal knowledge. The indigenous people of America refer to Quartz as the brain cells of Mother Earth, and this abundant crystal seems to instinctively know what is required. By attuning to your frequency, it transmutes negativity, amplifies energy, adjusts your vibrational field, and raises your consciousness. This deep soul cleanser removes the seeds of karmic dis-ease, detoxifies the emotional field, and balances your mind.

Quartz is silica, the most abundant element in the Earth and the human body.

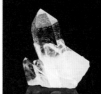

QUARTZ

Rhodochrosite

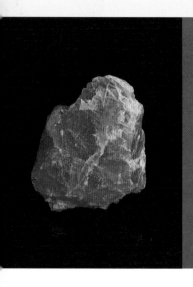

HARNESSING THE POWER

Program Rhodochrosite to attract
a twin flame, someone with whom
you can share unconditional love
and mutual support.

Rhodochrosite contains manganese, an important physiological constituent of the body with a powerful antioxidant and metabolic function.

THE POWER OF UNCONDITIONAL LOVE

Rose Quartz

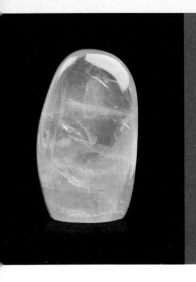

HARNESSING THE POWER

If you feel disempowered or unloved, hold Rose Quartz and remind yourself of a time when you felt positive and potent, loved and accepted.

TRANSFORMATIONAL POWER

During midlife crisis or traumatic times, Rose Quartz stabilizes emotions. It lets you look objectively at situations and keeps you from becoming emotionally overwhelmed. By dissolving guilt and bitterness, this crystal teaches you to love and accept yourself, forgive the past, and live from your heart. If you are unable to recognize where emotion is locked into your body, hold Rose Quartz, inhale deeply, and then exhale. Stay in the stillness of the out-breath and let your body tell you where it feels the tension. Breathe again to draw in healing love and direct it to the site with the power of your mind or by placing the crystal over the spot.

*Rose Quartz
heals emotions
and transforms
relationships with
yourself and others,
drawing in love
and harmony.*

ROSE QUARTZ

Sapphire

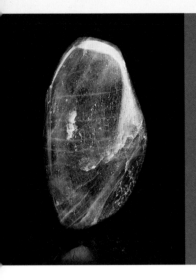

HARNESSING THE POWER

Wearing Sapphire reminds you that the soul is pure and innocent with perfect intention and moral integrity. It brings you peace of mind and serenity.

TRANSFORMATIONAL POWER

Sapphires come in many colors, and each has its own unique properties. Blue Sapphire encourages you to seek out spiritual truth. Pink Sapphire draws into your life exactly what you need to evolve. Yellow Sapphire is a crystal of abundance that attracts wealth and stimulates insight. Black Sapphire centers and protects. Star Sapphire provides you with a guiding star during the course of your life, supported by the three cross bars of faith, hope, and destiny.

*In the lapidaries of
the Middle Ages,
Sapphire was reputed
to heal the eyes, and
way back into history,
it was also used for
diseases of the blood.*

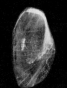

SAPPHIRE

Satyaloka™ & Satyamani™ Quartz

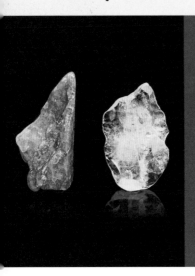

HARNESSING THE POWER

Placed on either side of your head, these Quartzes create an inner temple of light and facilitate direct communication with the divine.

TRANSFORMATIONAL POWER

Satyamani and Satyaloka Quartz effect enlightenment—quite literally. They bring light into the physical plane and open the illumined mind to an influx of pure spirit. These holy stones create an interface between the soul and the physical body, ensuring that you never walk your spiritual path alone.

These Quartzes work beyond the physical body to raise the frequencies of the subtle bodies and effect multidimensional, holistic soul healing.

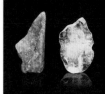

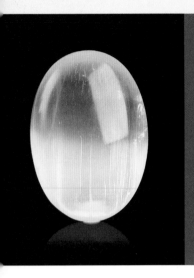

HARNESSING THE POWER

Hold Selenite above your head.
Feel it radiating divine light
through your whole being,
illuminating your inner temple
and connecting you to All That Is.

TRANSFORMATIONAL POWER

Selenite accesses angelic consciousness and brings divine light into everything it touches. White or Golden Selenite forms a bridge for the lightbody, facilitating expansion of consciousness and integration of the divine. A powerful transmutor for emotional energy, Selenite releases core feelings behind psychosomatic illnesses and emotional blockages. Connected to Persephone, Greek Queen of the Underworld, Peach Selenite shines light into dark places to help you understand your inner processes and integrate shadow qualities.

An eleventh-century lapidary says Selenite grows with the waxing moon and diminishes with the waning one.

SELENITE

Septarian

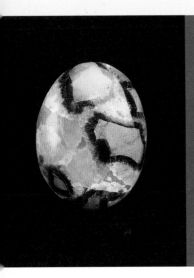

HARNESSING THE POWER

Keep a piece of Septarian with you when you speak in public—it helps you speak charismatically, with confidence and power.

If you speak in public, use Septarian to capture the audience's attention and let each person feel addressed individually.

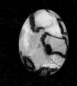

SEPTARIAN

Smoky Quartz

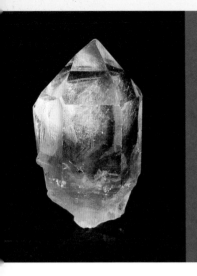

HARNESSING THE POWER

In a healing grid, Smoky Quartz absorbs disharmonious environmental energy. With the point facing out, it transmutes negative energy and with the point facing in, it draws in healing light.

TRANSFORMATIONAL POWER

Smoky Quartz's phenomenal power lies in its ability to transmute negative energies, purifying and returning them as core stability and energetic grounding. It is invaluable in healing layouts or for environmental healing. If your survival instincts are low, if you feel drained of energy or depleted by conditions around you, Smoky Quartz's psychological strength restores your vigor and shines light on the gifts that hide in the shadows of your inner being.

A large Smoky Quartz forms part of the Scepter of Power of the Scottish royal regalia.

SMOKY QUARTZ

Tiger's Eye

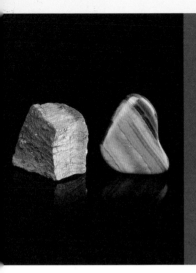

HARNESSING THE POWER

Grid Tiger's Eye or Hawk's Eye around your home to attract abundance and health. It also deflects anything that draws off or absorbs your abundance.

TRANSFORMATIONAL POWER

Tiger's Eye teaches integrity and right use of power. If you have misused, abused, or failed to take hold of your power in the past, this stone shows you how to let power flow through you for the good of all. If you are spaced out and uncommitted or overly proud and willful, wearing it develops your personal will assertively but sensitively. If you find it difficult to remain optimistic, particularly when things seem to be going well, carrying Tiger's Eye helps you trust in the future and set realistic goals for yourself. This stone balances your needs with others' and promotes creative compromise.

Traditionally, Tiger's Eye heals eye diseases and enhances night vision—it helps you see like a cat in the dark.

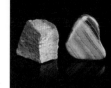

TIGER'S EYE

Topaz

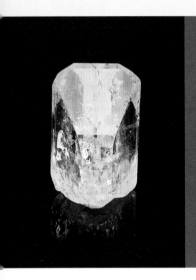

HARNESSING THE POWER

Wear Blue Topaz at your throat
to verbalize your feelings. It
connects to the angels of wisdom
and truth, and takes you into
interdimensional consciousness.

Topaz's power comes from its connection to the sun. Its name derives from the Sanskrit word for fire, which suggests its vibrant properties.

TOPAZ

Turquoise

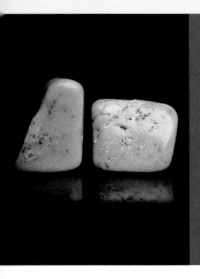

HARNESSING THE POWER

Placed over the throat chakra, Turquoise releases inhibitions and vows from the past that prevent you from fully expressing yourself.

An Arabic proverb states, "A turquoise given by a loving hand carries with it happiness and good fortune."

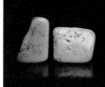

TURQUOISE

Zincite

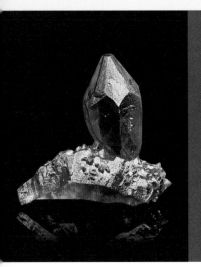

HARNESSING THE POWER

Placed over the base or sacral chakra, Zincite synthesizes personal power and creativity, empowering regeneration and manifestation on every level.

As suggested by the name, Zincite contains zinc, essential for cellular metabolism, teeth, bones, skin, and hair.

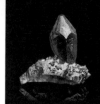

ZINCITE

Judy Hall is a successful Mind Body Spirit author with forty-two books to her credit including the million-selling *Crystal Bible (volumes 1 and 2)*. She has been a past-life therapist and karmic astrologer for more than forty years. An internationally known author, psychic, healer, broadcaster, and workshop leader, her books have been translated into fifteen languages. She recently appeared on the *Watkins Review* list of the one hundred most spiritually influential authors.

A trained healer and counselor, Judy has been psychic all her life and has a wide experience of many systems of divination and natural healing methods. Judy has a bachelor of education degree in religious studies with an extensive knowledge of world religions and mythology and a master of arts in cultural astronomy and astrology at Bath Spa University. Her mentor was Christine Hartley (Dion Fortune's metaphysical colleague and literary agent). She runs crystal, past life, and creative writing courses at her home in Dorset.

Her specialities are past-life readings and regression, soul healing, reincarnation, astrology and psychology, divination, and crystal lore. Judy has conducted workshops around the world and has made fifteen visits to Egypt, the subject of her novel *Torn Clouds*. See www.judyhall.co.uk.

Judy Hall would like to thank Robert Simmons of Heaven and Earth for permission to use the trademarked names designated™ within the text. John Van Rees Sr. and John Van Rees Jr. of Exquisite Crystals are to be congratulated for the wonderful crystal photography and have my gratitude for the introduction to Trigonics and many more marvelous crystals. I also bless David Eastoe of www.petaltone.co.uk, without whose cleansing, recharging, and ally essences I could not continue my crystal work. The translation of Theophrastus's work used throughout this book is by Earle R. Caley and John C. Richards, published by Columbia University, 1956. Their impeccable scholarship is to be applauded as it clarified nomenclature conundrums and highlighted false claims made by later "authorities." The Pliny translation is by D. E. Eichholz, Loeb Classical Library, and *The Lapidary of King Alfonso X The Learned*, by Ingrid Bahler and Katherine Gyekenyesi Gatto. *The Lithica* is taken from the 1864 (first) edition of Charles William King *The Natural History, Ancient and Modern, of Precious Stones and Gems, and of Precious Metals* (it was omitted from later editions). Over the past forty years plus, I have read several hundred books and articles, ancient and modern, about stones, their properties, history, and legends and cannot possibly acknowledge—or even remember—them all, but I thank everyone, especially my workshop participants, for their contribution to my knowledge. Heartfelt thanks also to Skye Alexander for her sensitive editing and thought-provoking questions.